D0591146

JULIAN MESSNER • NEW YORK

JEM

A JEM BOOK

Brush Up On Hair Care
Betty Lou Phillips

Illustrated by Lois Johnson

JULIAN MESSNER • NEW YORK

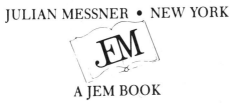

A JEM BOOK

Manufactured in the United States of America

Design by Stanley S. Drate

Library of Congress Cataloging in Publication Data

Phillips, Betty Lou.
   Brush up on hair care.

   "A Jem book."
   Includes index.
   Summary: Describes the physical structure of hair
and different hair types and discusses general
hair care including advice on shampooing, using the
proper tools, and choosing a hair style.
   1. Hair—Care and hygiene—Juvenile literature.
[1. Hair—Care and hygiene] I. Johnson, Lois, ill.
II. Title.
RL91.P48   1982   646.7′24   82-60643
ISBN 0-671-43852-2

Contents

Introduction   7

1   Inside Information   9

2   Get To Know Your Hair   16

3   Let Beauty Go To Your Head   23

4   Keep It Clean   27

5   How To Handle Your Hair   46

6   Shape Hair Up   55

7   Highlight Your Hair   63

8   Head in the Right Direction   69

9   Guard Against the Weather   71

Index   78

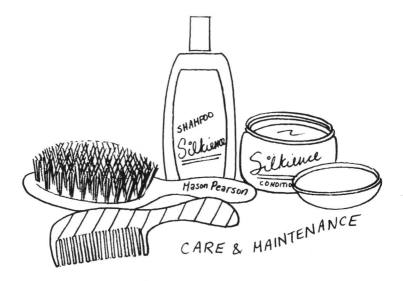

Products for good hair care and
maintenance.

Introduction

Are you happy with your hair? If you've ever said, "I can't do a thing with it," let that be a clue. Your hair needs some help.

Read on. We'll help you get to the root of your hair problem. Best of all, we'll show you how to have great-looking hair. Unless, of course, you already do. Then your aim is to keep it. The more you know about your hair, the easier this will be to do.

Hair that bounces and behaves doesn't just happen. Nature sets the texture and growth rate of your hair. All other traits depend largely on you. Your hair is only as healthy as you are. A proper diet, rest, and plenty of exercise all play a part in how your hair looks.

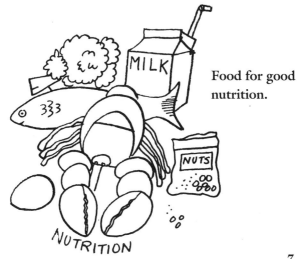

Food for good nutrition.

1

Inside Information

Your hair is often the first thing people look at when they meet you. When it looks good, you generally look good. You usually feel good, too. When you're happy with yourself, it shows. It shows that you take pride in yourself. What's more, when you look your best, you glow. Then somehow everything seems easier. It's easier to raise your hand in class, score points in sports, and even get a date for a big night. Think it over. Why not go ahead, and learn about your hair?

Anybody can have great hair. What's the secret? There is no secret. It's science—understanding the hair. After that, all you really need is a good haircut and good hair care habits. Then it's easy to get your hair to look its very best every day.

A Science Lesson

Your hair is mostly protein—97 percent, to be exact. The other 3 percent is water. The water comes from the air to which your hair is exposed. Too much moisture in the hair causes it to stretch and droop. Too little moisture makes hair brittle. Then it tends to split and break.

Parts of the Hair

Each slim strand of hair is made up of three layers: the *cuticle, cortex,* and *medulla.* All three must be in top shape for your hair to look its best.

The outer layer of the hair strand or shaft is called the *cuticle.* It is made up of tough, overlapping cells that protect the hair. These cells look somewhat like shingles on a roof. When the cuticle is in good shape, the cells lie flat and snug. Dirt can't enter. Moisture can't get out. So your hair has body and sheen.

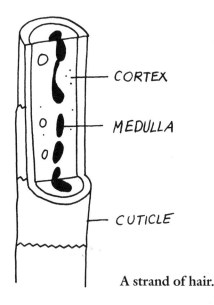

A strand of hair.

An overdose of either sun, wind, cold, or salt or chlorinated water, takes its toll on your hair. So does lots of tugging, curling, blow drying, and twisting. All these things can cause a strand of hair to swell. Then the cuticle rises up. Moisture escapes. Soon the hair looks frizzy, stringy, and dry.

The *cortex* is the middle layer of the hair shaft. It holds the pigment or *melanin* that gives hair color. Melanin is a black-brown pigment found in both skin and hair. It is scarce in honey blonds and people with auburn or red hair. Gray hair has no melanin at all. Your hair color is set at birth. Whether or not your hair turns gray one day depends mostly on your genes and how much melanin your body makes.

The *medulla* is the empty tube within the cortex. Scientists are not sure of its purpose.

At the Root of it All

The hair that you see on your head is dead! It has no nerves or blood supply. The living part of a hair is the *root*. It lies in a *follicle*—cavity—under the scalp. Many hair follicles close together produce a thick head of hair. People with a thin head of hair have fewer follicles, set further apart.

The shape of the follicle and the way your hair grows determines whether you have straight, wavy, or curly hair. Straight hair usually grows from a round hair shaft at an even rate. Wavy hair tends to sprout from an oval shaft. If you have curly hair, your hair shaft is nearly flat. Both waves and curls are caused by hair growing faster

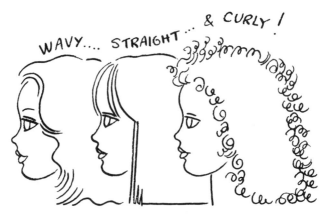

Types of hair.

on one side than the other. First, cells on one side of the follicle grow. Hair will bend that way. Then the other side produces cells, and hair will bend that way. So hair grows bent and wavy. The amount of curl you have can be changed only after the hair has grown out from the scalp.

At the sides of each follicle are *oil glands*. They keep hair from being stiff. They coat each strand and seal in moisture.

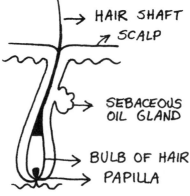

The root of a hair.

At the base of the follicle is the *papilla*. It has veins, arteries, and nerves. An artery carries blood to the root and nourishes it. If your body is poorly fed, your hair will suffer. For hair to grow healthy, a balanced diet is a must!

Did You Know . . . ?

There are over 100,000 hairs on the average head. The experts say those with black hair have about 108,000 strands. If your hair is brown, 109,000 is average. Blonds have the most strands on their heads—140,000. Redheads generally have the least—90,000. Red hairs, however, are the fattest of all. Blond hair shafts are the thinnest. So more blond hairs are needed to make up a full head of hair.

Some people's hair grows faster than others. But nearly everyone's hair grows faster in the summer than in the winter. Most hair grows about one-third of a millimeter a day, or about one-half inch a month. You grow about six inches of new hair a year. If you laid each strand of all the hair you grow in a year end-to-end, you would find that it totals almost eight miles.

Each hair grows, then rests, and then drops out or is pushed out by new hair. Usually 90 percent of the hairs on your head are growing at one time. The other 10 percent are resting. A hair's life cycle can last anywhere from two to six years. The longer the growing stage, the longer the hair. When a hair reaches the end of its life cycle, it falls out. Each hair is in a different stage of its life cycle. This explains why hair isn't all shed at the same time.

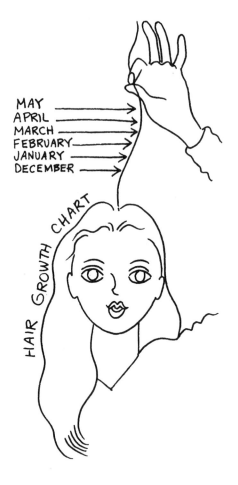

Most people lose between 50 and 250 hairs a day. For every "dropout," a new strand grows in its place. Don't panic if you see hair on your brush. You aren't going bald. If you do think you're losing more than your share, see a doctor. But first, think about how you treat your hair. Also, check if the hair you're losing is broken. Broken hair is usually the result of overbleaching or improper brushing.

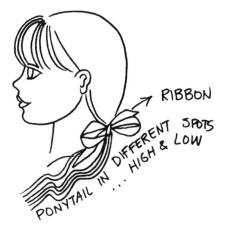

RIBBON

PONYTAIL IN ... DIFFERENT SPOTS HIGH & LOW

Secure a ponytail in different spots.

Wearing hair in a ponytail can also cause strain. (If you like to wear your hair back, make sure you don't always tie it back in the same place or tie it too tightly. Always use a coated elastic band. A rubber band causes breakage.)

Look at a hair carefully. If you see the hair root at one end, it's a "dropout."

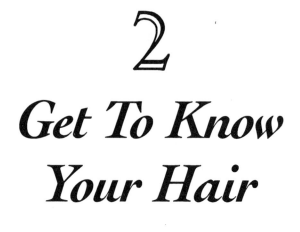

2

Get To Know Your Hair

Some types of hair need more care than others to get them looking their best. This means you've got to know your hair. Ask yourself some questions. If you can't pin down the answers, we'll help you out. Here's what you need to know.

• What type of hair do you have? Is it oily, dry, or normal? Perhaps it's a combination.

• What is its texture? Is it coarse, medium, or fine?

• How about its other qualities? Is your hair thick, thin, or in-between? Is it straight, curly, or wavy?

• Have you painted, bleached, streaked, colored, permed, or straightened your locks? If so, you have what's called processed hair.

Hair Type

If you have doubts about your hair type, check the telltale signs below. Pick the type that most closely matches your hair.

OILY. A set won't hold. It wilts, leaving hair hanging limply. Hair looks stringy if it is not shampooed daily. When hair has the stringies, chances are it also has a case of the greasies. This is a buildup of extra oil on the scalp that works its way through the hair. That's why strands tend to clump together. Often, oily hair goes together with an itchy scalp. The scalp may even be flaky at times.

Does this sound like your hair? During the teen years, changes in the body can cause the scalp's oil glands to produce too much oil. Your period and stress

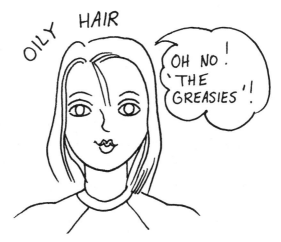

Oily hair looks stringy.

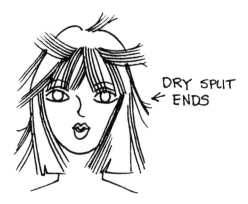

**Dry hair has lots of static electricity
when brushed.**

make matters worse. Oil also draws dirt. All of this can cause you and your hair to droop.

DRY. Dull hair usually means dry hair. Hair that's frizzy and feels like a haystack is also dry. Dry hair splits and breaks easily. It has lots of static electricity when combed or brushed. This makes it hard to manage. Dry hair lacks holding power when set. On the good side, hair that's dry can go days without needing shampooing.

Dull, dry, flyaway hair that tends to break off easily often comes from "too much" of something. There is too much heating, bleaching, perming, or straightening. Only in a few cases is dry hair inherited. When the scalp's oil glands fail to replace oil that's lost, hair becomes dry.

NORMAL. This is hair that's neither oily nor dry. Instead, it's alive with body and has a strong, healthy look. Anyone with normal hair is truly fortunate.

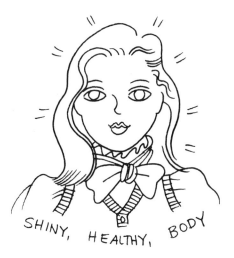

SHINY, HEALTHY, BODY

Healthy, normal hair.

COMBINATION. Many people have some combination of the above. For example, you may have dry ends and oily roots.

Hair Texture

COARSE. Hair that's coarse feels wiry and may be difficult to manage. In good condition, each strand is strong and fat. Coarse hair usually grows outward, rather than down. That's why it's nearly impossible to force coarse hair into a smooth style unless it is covered with setting gel.

FINE. Fine hair feels baby soft and silky. But it often lacks body. It may not hold a set well. Also, fine hair often has lots of static electricity which makes it look flyaway.

19

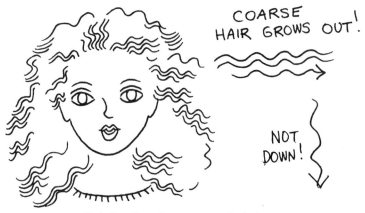

It is hard to force coarse hair into a smooth style.

MEDIUM. This is hair that's neither coarse nor fine. Because it's somewhere in-between, it is usually easy to manage.

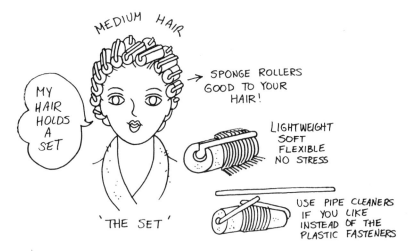

Medium hair is easy to manage.

Hair Qualities

Few of us are *really* happy with our lot. If we have straight hair, we wish it was curly. We often pay a fortune to have curls. Those with curly hair spend a lot of money to go straight. As for color, almost everyone thinks blondes have more fun. At some time, most women consider going blond—or adding highlights to liven up their hair.

But you can't turn fine hair into coarse. You can't turn thin into thick or vice versa. Some conditioners claim to make hair thicker. What they really do is fill in spaces on the hair shaft. This gives a thicker look. What you can do is make the most of what you've got. Once you know what you have to work with, there's no reason to ever be hassled by your hair.

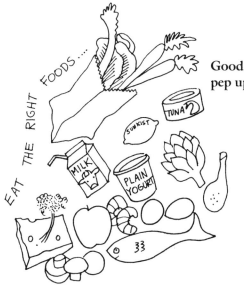

Good eating habits will pep up thin hair.

THIN. Thin hair can be coarse, fine, or in-between. There just isn't a lot of it. This is often because the follicles are spaced far apart on the scalp. Thin hair can also be caused by stress or too much tugging and twisting. Crash diets can cause hair to thin, too. But hair condition quickly improves when eating habits do.

THICK. Many follicles set close together produce a thick head of hair. Lift your hair at the forehead and check. Here's something else to notice: the coarser a hair, the more space it takes up on the scalp.

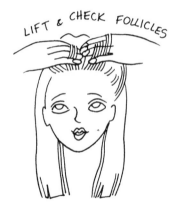

Processed Hair

If your hair has been permed, painted, colored, bleached, or straightened, its makeup has been changed. Any chemical treatment alters the hair. What's more, chemicals can be damaging if not properly applied. (For more about processing, see page 45.)

3

Let Beauty Go To Your Head

We all want to look good. *Nothing* adds to our looks as much as good-looking hair. Furthermore, the best-looking hair is clean hair. If your hair isn't clean, all the styling in the world won't help!

How often you need to shampoo depends on your hair type. It also depends on where you live and how active you are. If your hair is oily, you'll need to shampoo more often than a friend with dry or normal hair. If you live in the city, you'll have to lather up more often too. Fumes from cars and buses can cause hair to get dirtier faster. You won't need to wash your hair nearly as often if you live in the country.

No matter where you live, you'll need to shampoo more in the summer than in the winter. Hot weather makes you perspire. Perspiration makes hair sticky, and damp hair draws dirt. When you're active in sports, you need to shower more often. You need to suds your hair more too.

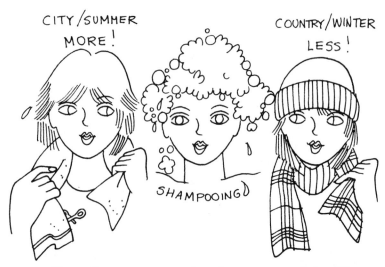

How often you may need to shampoo your hair will depend on where you live and what season it is.

Shampoo as often as necessary. If you use a mild shampoo, even a daily sudsing won't harm your hair. Dry hair results from washing too often with a harsh shampoo. That's one that strips the hair of moisture.

A good shampoo cleans hair quickly and then easily rinses out. It's gentle. It leaves your hair easy to handle and smelling good too.

Be Picky

With so many shampoos to choose from, finding the best one can be a task. You must know which product suits you. You also need to know how to shampoo. These are the keys to making your hair do what *you* want it to.

No one shampoo is right for everybody. The one that is best for you depends on your hair. Most shampoos are made specifically for oily, dry, or normal hair. The difference is in the amount of soap. The oily mixture has more soap as oily hair attracts more grime. Shampoo for dry hair has less soap. The drier the hair is, the milder the formula it needs. Colored or damaged hair demands the gentlest shampoo of all.

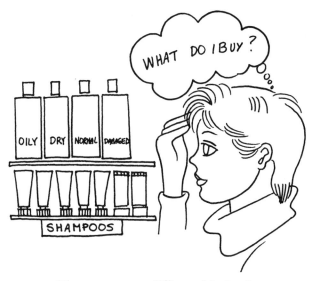

There are many different kinds of shampoo.

Don't make the mistake of thinking that baby shampoos are best for hair. The big plus of baby shampoos is that they don't sting the eyes. But just because a shampoo is easy on the eyes, that doesn't mean it's better for hair.

Hair is mostly protein. Shampoos with protein added to them help put life into hair. They protect all types of hair by sealing the cuticle.

Use a protein-rich shampoo that matches your hair type and is geared to its needs. After that, finding the shampoo that's just right for you is really a matter of trial and error. To test the shampoo first, buy a small size. Once you've found a good shampoo, there's no need to switch brands. Why mess with success? If a shampoo is doing the job for you, continue using it. Change brands only if there's a change in your hair's needs. (See Weather, page 71.)

4

Keep It Clean

Y ou may be washing your hair several times a week. But are you sure you're doing it the best way? Here's the proper way to shampoo. First, carefully brush out all tangles. Brushing also loosens dirt. Shampooing in the shower makes rinsing easy. If a shower isn't handy, bend over a tub. Then wet your hair *thoroughly* with warm water. Very hot water can burn the scalp and damage hair.

Pour a little shampoo into your hands. Never apply soap directly to the hair. The shampoo will wind up all in one spot. One capful is usually plenty for short hair. Two capfuls is good for hair that's long and thick. Read the directions on the back of the shampoo bottle. Be sure to follow them.

Work up a good lather. Wash the hair from front to back. Use the pads of your fingertips to gently massage the scalp. Don't use your nails or you may hurt your head. Remember, you're not shampooing just to have clean hair. You want a clean scalp too. That's why it's important to work the soap in well. Shampoo from the scalp to the very ends of the hair. Don't forget about shampooing your hairline.

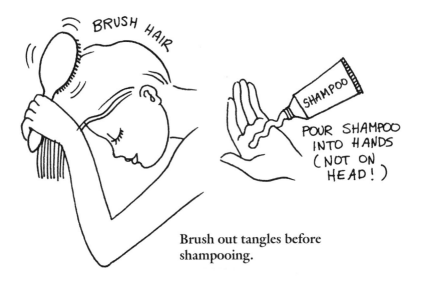

Brush out tangles before shampooing.

Rinse hair with warm water. One shampoo is all that's needed if you wash your hair daily. If you don't, suds hair again. Then rinse well.

Always shampoo carefully. Hair is weakest when it's wet. To prevent tangling and damaging your hair, don't

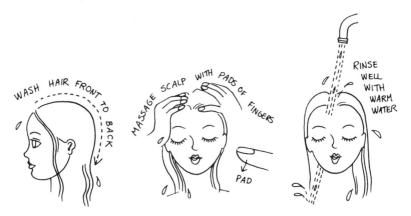

pile long hair on top of your head. Be sure to rinse all shampoo out. Leftover soap dulls hair. Even when you're sure you've rinsed enough, rinse once again. Finish with a cool water rinse. This will leave your hair extra shiny. Then gently squeeze water from the hair.

Hair Helpers

Follow your shampoo with a creme rinse, if you're short on time. Otherwise a conditioner is even better.

Creme rinses leave just-shampooed hair shiny, soft, and easy to comb. Less tugging means less chance of harming hair. Creme rinses also coat the cuticle with a slippery film. This helps do away with flyaway hair.

For best results, never use too much creme rinse. It's also a good idea to comb the creme rinse through your hair. As you rinse, untangle strands with your fingers. Unless you rinse very well, hair is apt to be droopy.

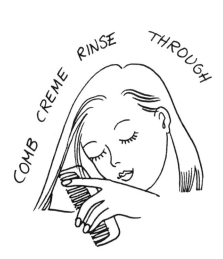

A creme rinse tames hair that's dry or bushy. Using one on oily hair may make the hair limp. However, even oily hair needs a creme rinse on dry ends at times.

It would be grand if a creme rinse could improve your hair's condition. It can't. Only a good conditioner can do that.

Hair that's in top condition is glossy, sleek, and manageable. Hair that's in bad shape lacks luster, body, and bounce. It also tangles and breaks easily. It is dry and hard to manage.

You'd be surprised if you looked at a hair under a microscope. Damaged hair looks rutted and ragged like the drawings below. Do you see why hair like this would easily become tangled and be difficult to work with?

Give your hair the stretch test. Find out if your hair is ailing or well. Here's how it's done. Pull about six sample hairs from your head. Take them from different

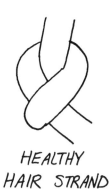

HEALTHY
HAIR STRAND

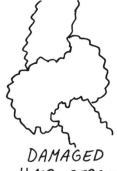

DAMAGED
HAIR STRAND

spots. Then wrap the hairs around two fingers and pull. Does your hair break easily? If it does, it doesn't have much stretch. That means it needs a well-planned conditioning program.

Weekly instant conditioning will keep hair with give manageable. A monthly deep conditioning treatment will give it an added boost.

Instant conditioners smooth the cuticle. They give even dull hair sheen in no time flat. The best conditioners do more than help hair reflect light. They add body. And everyone knows, hair with added body will hold a better set.

If you have dried-out, mistreated hair, instant conditioning is not enough. Your hair needs *extra* help to bounce back. *Deep conditioners* fill the bill. Deep conditioners are rich in protein. They fill in open spaces, seal the cuticle, and trap moisture for shine. Ailing hair may need a deep conditioning treatment once a week. Normal hair needs it about once a month. Oily hair rarely needs a deep conditioning treatment.

Look for a conditioner that's designed for your type of hair. You can even pick a natural conditioner. Look in the refrigerator. There are three good choices: an egg, honey, and mayonnaise.

The nice thing is that all are cheap and easy to use. Make sure your hair is shiny clean. Towel dry it. Then rub raw egg (or three to four tablespoons of honey or mayonnaise) down the hair shafts with your fingers. Comb it through. There's no need to massage the conditioner into your scalp.

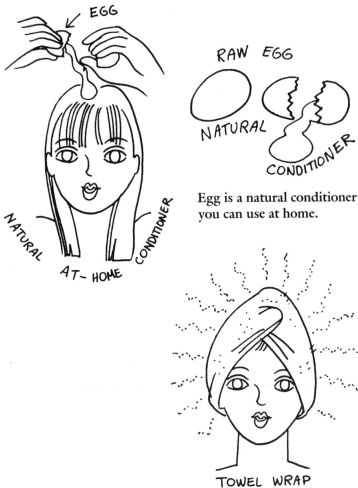

RAW EGG

NATURAL CONDITIONER

Egg is a natural conditioner you can use at home.

NATURAL AT-HOME CONDITIONER

TOWEL WRAP CONDITIONING

Leave the conditioner on for an hour or more. It takes time for a deep conditioner to work. Heat can speed things up. It causes the cells of the cuticle to lift and open up. This makes it easy for the conditioner to get inside the hair shaft.

Wrap your head in a warm, damp towel or clip a plastic bag over your hair, but not over your face. Sit in a warm spot. The bathtub's perfect. Relax, while you read. Or pamper yourself, if you prefer. Put the sparkle back in your eyes after a day at the beach. Remove all eye makeup. Lie back and put potato slices on your closed eyelids. Think cool thoughts for at least fifteen minutes. When the time is up, remove the potato slices, and shampoo the conditioner out. You may need two shampoos. Then rinse with warm water.

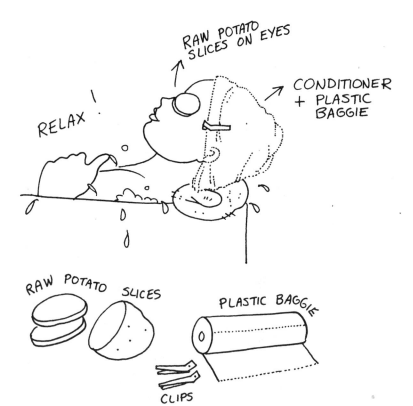

RAW POTATO SLICES ON EYES

CONDITIONER + PLASTIC BAGGIE

RELAX!

RAW POTATO SLICES

PLASTIC BAGGIE

CLIPS

Next, towel-pat your hair dry. Don't rub it with the towel. You'll wind up with a tangled mess. Finally, gently comb your hair.

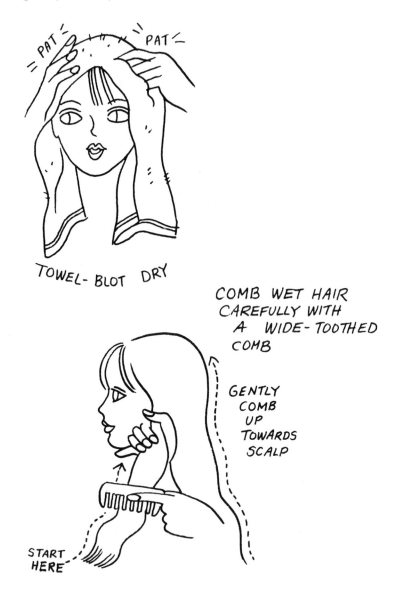

PAT

PAT

TOWEL- BLOT DRY

COMB WET HAIR CAREFULLY WITH A WIDE-TOOTHED COMB

GENTLY COMB UP TOWARDS SCALP

START HERE

Now Hear This

Never brush wet hair. When hair is wet, it's stretched to its full length. Like a stretched-out rubber band, it's easily damaged. Brushing can cause wet hair to break. Instead of brushing, comb hair with a wide-tooth comb. Start at hair ends and work up inch by inch toward the scalp.

Parting Words

Always wash your comb and brush every time you shampoo. Do not use dirty tools on clean hair. First, clean your brush. Rake away the hair caught in the bristles with a comb. Then swish your brush gently in warm, soapy water until it is clean.

Don't use harsh soaps. Don't soak your brush. This can loosen bristles and damage a wooden handle. Rinse the brush in warm water and then shake the water off. Dry the brush with the bristles down on a clean, dry towel. Never dry the bristles with a towel. Never dry the brush over heat. Heat can harm the bristles.

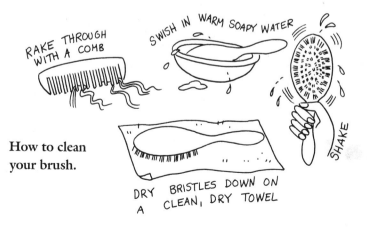

RAKE THROUGH WITH A COMB

SWISH IN WARM SOAPY WATER

SHAKE

How to clean your brush.

DRY BRISTLES DOWN ON A CLEAN, DRY TOWEL

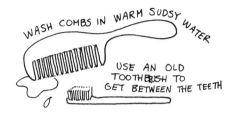

How to clean your comb.

Clean your comb in warm, sudsy water. Use an old toothbrush to get between the teeth. Then rinse well.

Afterwards, inspect your hair equipment. Frayed brushes, toothless combs, bent clips, and bobby pins without rubber tips all belong in the garbage. They can harm your hair.

First-Aid Tips

There are ways to correct your hair problems. Here are some step-by-step tips.

OILY HAIR. Finding the right shampoo is a must. Suds that are too harsh can strip your hair of oil. Oil glands then work overtime pouring out even more oil. This makes oily hair oilier. So shop around for the proper shampoo. Also:

- Shampoo daily.
- Finish with a lemon rinse (3 tablespoons lemon juice to 1 cup cool water).

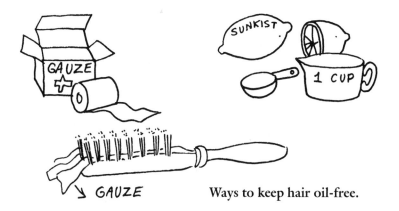

Ways to keep hair oil-free.

- Condition dry ends, not your whole head.
- Between shampoos, pad the rows of your brush bristles with gauze. Doing this will help absorb oil and dirt.
- Be sure that you're eating three balanced meals a day.
- Figure out what you can do to lower stress. Stress often makes oil glands overproduce.

DRY HAIR. If you're always frustrated because your hair is dry:
- Cut down on the number of times you shampoo.
- Try switching to a milder formula shampoo.
- Give your hair one instead of two sudsings.
- Follow with a vinegar rinse ($1/2$ cup vinegar to 2 cups cool water).
- Treat your hair to extra deep-conditioning.
- Keep hair covered outdoors. Most outdoor sports tend to make dry hair drier.
- Improve your diet. Try to use less salt.

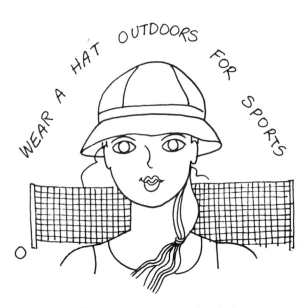

WEAR A HAT OUTDOORS FOR SPORTS

One way to protect dry hair.

- To add body and sheen, give your hair a warm oil bath before your next shampoo. (It's well worth the trouble and can't harm the hair.)

Follow these directions to give yourself an oil bath. Warm up about one-half cup of olive oil. Part your hair down the middle. With a cotton ball dab oil on your part and down the strands. Part hair inch by inch across the scalp. Repeat. When all the oil is used, comb hair to spread the oil evenly. Wrap hair in an old towel. Sit under a warm hair dryer for thirty to forty minutes. Then shampoo until the oil is all washed out. It'll take at least two good washings to rid your hair of the oil.

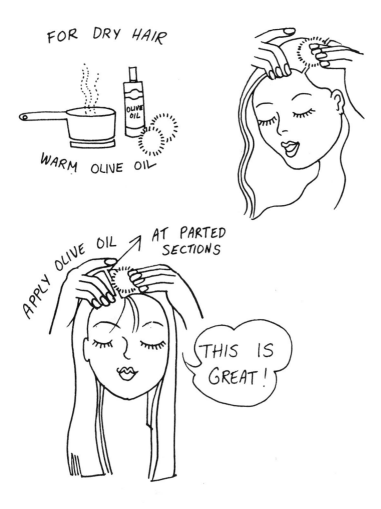

COMBINATION HAIR. Hair that's part oily, part dry needs special attention:

- Use a dry-hair shampoo one day, an oily-hair shampoo the next. Or, better yet, first use a dry shampoo on ends. Follow up with a shampoo for oily hair for the rest of your hair.
- Do the same with conditioners.

- Use a new shampoo on the market that says it's "self-adjusting." Read labels. Find a shampoo that says it cleans and conditions according to the needs of your hair.

THIN HAIR. To give your crop the look of fullness:
- Keep your hair super clean.
- Use a body-building, protein-rich shampoo.
- Let blow-drying lift your hair. (See page 50 for the how-to's.)
- Choose a short or medium cut.

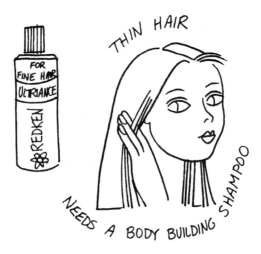

DANDRUFF. What you think is dandruff may be the result of sunburn, setting lotion, hair spray, or not rinsing your hair well. All can cause dandruff-like flakes.

True dandruff consists of dead skin cells clumped together. The skin is forever forming new cells. As old

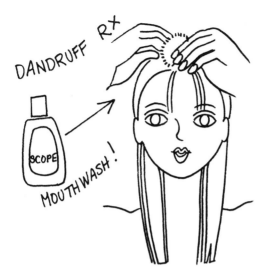

One way to take care of dandruff.

cells reach the surface, they die and fall off. These cells are generally so small you can't see them. Dandruff appears when oil and dead skin cells stick together.

How do you tell the difference between dandruff and other dead cell flakes? Flaking with red, itchy patches usually means true dandruff.

In any case, flakes of dead skin in your hair and on your shoulders are unsightly. Although experts don't know what really causes dandruff, here's how they suggest you attack the problem:

- Take a look at your diet.
- Try a dandruff or medicated shampoo. Use every other time you shampoo until the flakes are gone.
- Try this. Mix one part of any mouthwash with two parts warm water. Dab on scalp with a cotton ball.

The easiest way is to part hair inch by inch across the scalp, front to back, and dab along parts. Leave on for thirty minutes. Shampoo out.

- Avoid using setting lotions and hair sprays that can build up on the hair and scalp.
- Don't always part your hair in the same place. There'll be less chance of the sun burning your head.
- See your doctor if the problem doesn't clear up.

SPLIT ENDS. The careless use of hot rollers, curling irons, pressing combs, and blow dryers can cause a headful of split ends. Too much dye or bleach and too much brushing and teasing can also cause split ends. The only way to get rid of split ends and keep them from inching up the hair shaft is:

- Cut them off.
- Have your hair trimmed every six to eight weeks.
- Watch how you treat your hair.

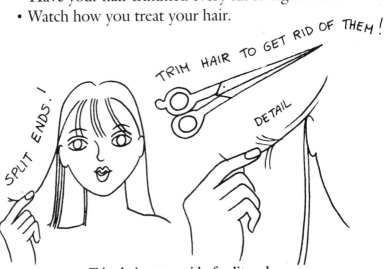

Trim hair to get rid of split ends.

BLACK HAIR. Most blacks have naturally curly hair. Many people even have kinky hair. Kinky hair tends to be thick in some spots and thin in others. That's why it tends to get twisted and tangled up. Tangles make any hair hard to comb and likely to break easily. The curlier hair is, the harder it is for scalp oil to reach the ends. As a result, black hair is especially prone to dryness. (This is why it seldom needs daily shampooing.) Furthermore, light is spread every which way when it hits curly hair. So your hair may lack luster.

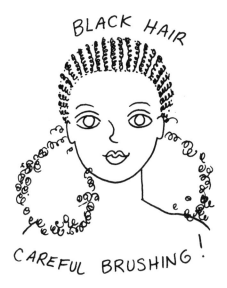

BLACK HAIR

CAREFUL BRUSHING!

What should you do? Take note of all that you read in this book. Remember also that black hair needs products all its own for more shine and manageability. In addition:

- A weekly shampoo is a must. Try a good protein shampoo, perhaps one for dry hair. Massage your scalp well as you wash.
- Follow the shampoo with a detangler.
- Treat hair to a deep conditioner once or twice a month. Avoid conditioners that simply coat the hair. What's best for you are those that can be absorbed by the hair shaft. When conditioning your hair, don't forget the product needs time to work!
- Be very careful when styling your hair. Towel dry it first. Comb and brush it carefully. Blow-drying may make your hair bushy. Don't use sponge rollers for your set. They tend to dry out the hair.
- Straighten only new growth, not previously straightened hair.
- Use a brush with soft bristles or one with round, rubber teeth.

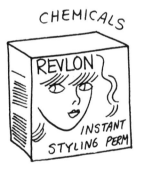

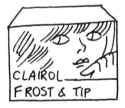

PROCESSED HAIR. When your hair needs help fast, it's smart to let a pro take over. Why cause more trouble, especially if you've fooled with Mother Nature and now have green hair. For HOTLINE HELP, call CLAIROL, toll free. Dial 1-800-223-5800. In New York State, call collect 1-212-644-2990.

5

How To Handle Your Hair

Do you wish you had terrific-looking hair? Who doesn't! Simply wishing isn't enough, however. How your hair looks depends mostly on you. That doesn't mean you must spend lots of money at the hairdresser's, or hours under a dryer. What it takes to get the look you're aiming for is just plain practice. So go ahead, practice working with your hair.

Basic Tools

For starters, two basic tools are needed. A wide-toothed comb with smooth, *round* tips for removing tangles is a must. A good hairbrush for styling is also necessary. Squared or pointed comb teeth can hurt the scalp and split the hair. When teeth are set wide, it's easier for a comb to get through the hair without pulling. A plastic comb is a good choice.

A good brush is your hair's best friend. It can make a big difference in the way your hair looks. Finding the right brush takes some know-how.

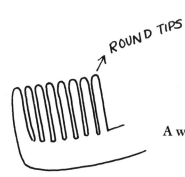

ROUND TIPS

A wide-toothed comb.

Choose the Proper Brush for the Job

Say good-bye to the frizzies. For hair that's sleek and smooth, pick a brush with natural bristles. Brushes come with three different types of bristles—natural, synthetic (nylon), and a mixture of both.

Natural bristles are the best. They hold moisture. This helps spread scalp oils through the hair for a

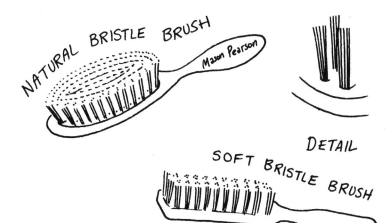

NATURAL BRISTLE BRUSH

Mason Pearson

DETAIL

SOFT BRISTLE BRUSH

healthy shine. Nylon doesn't do this. Natural bristles also separate hair strands. This helps add bulk to hair. With proper care a good bristle brush will last at least five years. It is worth the money to buy one.

Look for bristles of varying lengths with rounded ends. They don't scratch the scalp or tear at the hair. Never use a brush with sharp bristles.

Those bristles set in rubber have added give. This keeps them from tugging at the hair. A brush with a rubber base can also reduce static electricity.

The texture of your hair counts in choosing a brush. The coarser and thicker your hair, the stiffer the bristles should be. Otherwise they may not reach the roots. Then brushing won't do hair much good. Select a soft bristle brush for long, thin, fine, or permed hair to avoid hair stretching or breaking.

Do It Right

Just brushing your hair isn't enough. Doing a good job is important. Brushing properly wakes up the scalp. It picks up any dirt and at the same time it spreads oil through hair. Before you brush your hair, loosen tangles and knots with a comb.

Here's the way to brush. Stand up. Bend from the waist. Toss hair forward so it hangs down in front of your face. Start at the back of your head. If you have short hair, brush out from the scalp to ends in slow, firm strokes. If your hair is long, brush down to your ears. Then hold hair at this spot with your free hand and

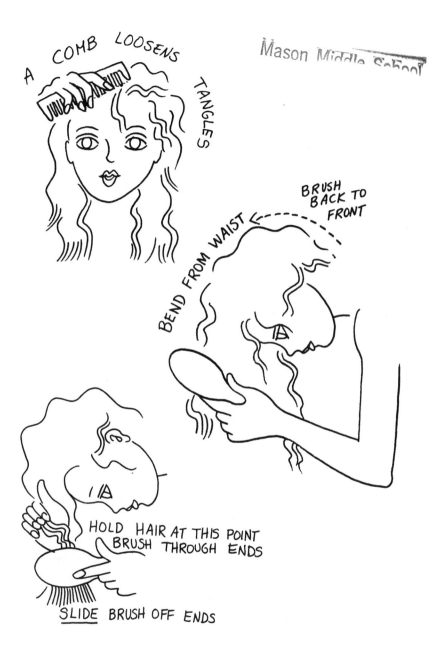

The how-tos of correct brushing.

run the brush through ends. For your hair's sake, finish off each stroke by *sliding* the brush off the ends.

Never brush long hair in one long stroke. This puts too much strain on both hair and roots. *Always* brush gently. If you brush too harshly, you may break your hair. Be sure to brush your entire head. Then stand up. Toss your head back and brush hair into place.

Forget that myth about brushing 100 strokes a day. That's too much stress for most hair. What's more, too much brushing starts oil glands pumping. You don't want oily hair. Just brush enough to keep hair well groomed.

Use a wide-toothed comb on wet hair. Begin at ends and work toward the roots. If you run into a tangle, loosen it gently with your fingers. Then continue combing. Don't tug at a tangle. When you jerk out snarls you're snapping hairs and splitting ends.

Blow-Drying

Let your hair air dry if you can. It takes a little longer, but it's easier on the hair. The daily use of a hair blower can damage hair. This is especially true if the dryer is set on high. When you're short on time, set the blow dryer on medium. If your hair is dry or fine, keep it set at low.

For the best results, bend over and comb your hair forward. Starting at the nape of the neck, begin drying your hair. Hold the dryer at least six inches from your head. To avoid drying out hair, keep the dryer moving. Lift hair with your fingers to help hair dry. This also helps guide hair into shape.

50

How to blow dry your hair.

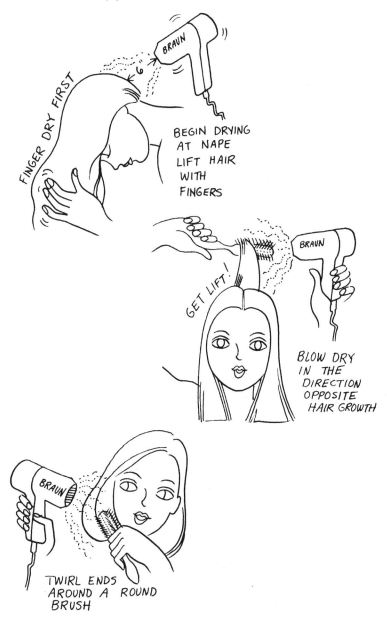

FINGER DRY FIRST

BRAUN

BEGIN DRYING
AT NAPE
LIFT HAIR
WITH
FINGERS

GET LIFT!

BRAUN

BLOW DRY
IN THE
DIRECTION
OPPOSITE
HAIR GROWTH

BRAUN

TWIRL ENDS
AROUND A ROUND
BRUSH

Treat hair gently. Never pull or tug at it while drying. Don't try to style soaking-wet hair. After a shampoo, dry hair until it's just damp. A round, natural bristle brush is perfect for turning ends under.

To style, divide hair into sections. Secure with clips. Work section by section. Blow dry bottom layers at back first. Hold the brush in one hand, the dryer in the other. Follow the brush with the dryer.

Blow dry *opposite* the natural growth of the hair. This will keep strands from clinging to the head. It will also blow in fullness. To get lift all over, finish drying the roots first. Twirl ends on the brush and lift hair high. Dry. Then roll hair all the way to the roots. Hold and dry. Now slowly unwind the brush. Clip freshly curled hair out of the way and repeat.

Curling Cues

Hot rollers and curling irons can put more curl into hair than a blow dryer. But they aren't for daily use. This is especially so if hair is fine, dry, or thin. Both steal moisture from hair. Hair has little to begin with—and none to spare.

Never heat dirty hair. You'll scorch the cuticle. Also, be careful to keep a hot curling wand barrel away from the scalp.

Another tip: Don't sleep in rollers. They break and pull hair.

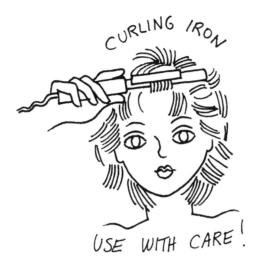

CURLING IRON

USE WITH CARE!

Ready To Roll

When your hair looks just plain "blah," the fastest way to add curl is with hot rollers. Always follow the directions for use. And . . .

• Make sure hair is dry.

• Use a wide-toothed comb to section hair. Clip in place.

• Select rollers with care. The larger the section wrapped around the roller, the tighter the curl. The roller size also makes a difference. In general, a roller gives a curl about twice as large as it is. The bigger the roller, the softer the curl. So the tighter the curl you want, the smaller the roller should be. If curls are too tight, put more hair on each roller.

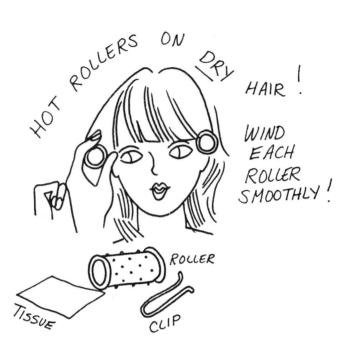

How to set your hair with hot rollers.

• Protect hair by putting tissue around the bottom of each section of hair before you roll it up.

• Gently stretch hair as you wind. Don't pull.

• Wind all rollers neatly to get a smooth set. If hair ends aren't wrapped smoothly around rollers, they'll look like fish hooks when set.

• For a tight set, leave rollers in until they're cool. The longer you leave them in, the tighter the curl.

• All set? To help prevent tangling, unroll slowly. Remove bottom rollers first. Work up.

• Let hair cool before brushing or you'll brush out the set!

6

Shape Hair Up

Tired of wearing your hair the same old way? Like the look of a style that's new? When you're also spending too much time fussing with your hair—washing, drying, curling, crimping—it's time for a change! Hair should be easy to care for—whether it's short or long.

You probably look good in lots of hair styles. Naturally, some look better on you than others. The shape of your face has a lot to do with the way your hair looks best. If you're not sure about your face shape, do this. Tie hair back and look into the bathroom mirror. With a piece of soap, carefully draw on the mirror the outline of your face. Step back. Match the shape you've drawn with the drawings here. (Clean off the mirror!)

To help you find a new style that flatters your face, here are a few hints.

OVAL. If you have an oval face, you're lucky. You can wear any hair style—long, short, straight, curly. You're the one the center part was made for. (The exception to this is if you have a large nose. Then a

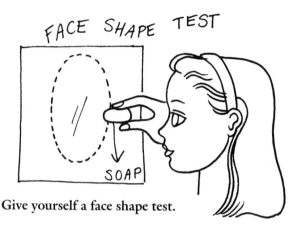

Give yourself a face shape test.

center part will become an arrow pointing at your nose. Straight bangs also will call attention to its size.) But do try whatever suits your fancy. Your face is the perfect shape.

SQUARE. Play down a broad forehead with wispy, side-swept bangs. Roll the rest of your hair under in a chin-length pageboy. Hair that moves will distract from your squarish jaw. Adding fullness at your jawline will also emphasize your eyes and cheekbones.

SQUARE

HEART. Do you have a wide forehead? How about a narrow chin? Choose a mix of smooth and fluffy. Brush hair smooth and close to head at crown, temples, and sides. Let a soft, full flip add width to your chin.

HEART

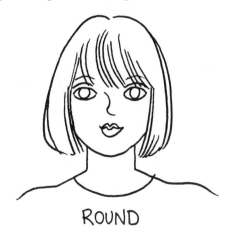

ROUND. Avoid any hairdo that's brushed back. It'll only make you look like a "dumpling" face. Stick to a soft style that frames the face. Draw eyes to the top of your head by adding a little height there.

ROUND

PEAR. A face that's wide at the bottom and narrow at the top needs fullness on top and at the sides. Think curly and short.

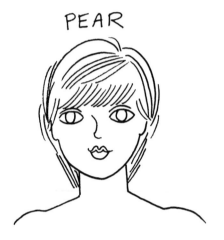

PEAR

OBLONG. Opt for fullish hair that frames the face with long, feathery bangs on the forehead. This will make your long face seem fuller.

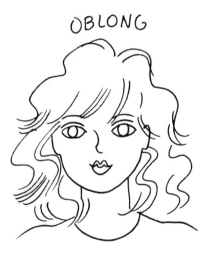

OBLONG

DIAMOND. Frame the face at the temples and chin, keeping hair close to the head at the widest points. Bangs and a chin-length pageboy can do wonders for your looks.

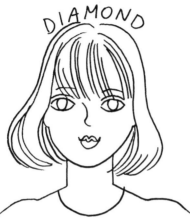

Take A Short Cut

You know what you want. A new haircut that suits your face, hair type, and you! One that makes you feel good—every day! You also want a few ideas for different ways to wear the same basic cut.

You also know what you don't want. You don't want hair in your eyes. You don't want a fussy hairdo. You also don't want one that doesn't flatter you, even if it is the latest fad.

A bad haircut is forever. It certainly seems that way if you've ever had one. Chances are by now you have. That's why just thinking about getting your hair trimmed can be scary. But it can be less so, if you heed the following tips.

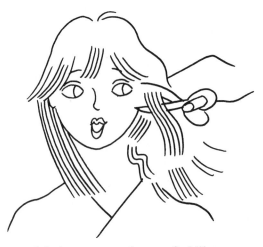

A haircut can make you feel like a new person.

Have a professional hair stylist cut your hair. It's worth the money. Shop around. Don't call just any beauty salon and take any hair stylist available. If you know a haircutter whose work you like, great. Set up an appointment. Otherwise, ask a friend with terrific-looking hair for the name of her hairdresser. Write a major chain for recommendations. For instance, Seligman & Latz (666 Fifth Avenue, New York 10019) or Glemby (120 E. 16th Street, New York 10003). Tell them a little about yourself and your hair.

When you make an appointment, ask that it start with a consultation or talk. Tell the hair stylist about yourself. Mention sports you enjoy. Tell how handy you are with your hair. Also share with her or him any hair problems you're having, or have had in the past. Take out any pictures you've collected of the hairdo you want. Let the hair stylist know how much time you have to spend on your hair.

Then listen to the hair stylist. Consider his or her advice. Sometimes what looks great on someone else isn't really right for you. Hair looks best when you don't fight the way it grows, its texture, or its movement. You don't want to wind up having a daily battle with your hair. A good hair stylist can guide you in your choice.

Before the haircut gets underway, make sure you and the hair stylist agree. See that you understand what the finished cut will look like. Will it be short? How short? Long? How long? If there's *anything* you don't understand, be sure to ask. Shorter hair than you're ready for can be very upsetting.

If you and the hair stylist can't agree, offer to pay for the consultation. There's usually no charge. There's never a charge for a consultation if you go ahead and have the work done.

Showing the hair stylist a picture can help you get the haircut you want.

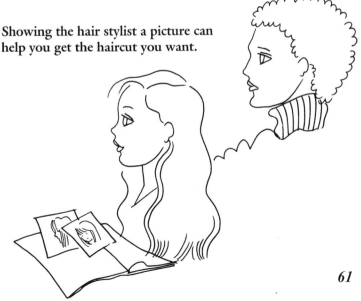

What happens if you still hate your hairdo afterwards? Don't panic. A cut often appeals more after you've gotten used to it. You should let your hair stylist know you're unhappy. Maybe there's something he or she can do.

Are you pleased with your hair? Don't leave the salon without letting the stylist know. Also be sure you've found out how to care for your hair between visits. Most haircuts hold their shape for six to eight weeks.

Tips on Tipping

Tip your hair stylist 15 percent of the bill. Give the person who shampoos your hair 75 cents or one dollar. In a New York salon, tip slightly more. No matter where you are, when the owner of a salon does your hair, no tip is expected.

The quickest way to figure a tip on, for example, a $15 bill, is take 10 percent of the amount ($1.50). Then halve it ($.75) and add up the two figures for the total tip.

7

Highlight Your Hair

*T*hinking of playing with Mother Nature? There are several ways of changing your hair color. Here are the most common.

TEMPORARY COLORING. This shampoos in. It washes out with the next sudsing. It contains no peroxide (bleach). It can't change your natural color. It can improve it by adding depth and highlights. This is a good way to take the brassiness out of bleached hair. It can also add life to hair that's mousey brown.

SEMIPERMANENT COLORING. This shampoos in, but is somewhat stronger than temporary coloring. It doesn't have to be applied after every shampoo. Because it is left on for a short while, the color sinks into the hair shaft. It cannot lighten hair since it contains no bleach. It can brighten and bolster color. This type of coloring lasts for three or four shampoos.

PERMANENT COLORING. This contains peroxide that can lighten hair up to three shades lighter than your own. If you want hair that's lighter than that, it's a two-step process. It can also color hair darker. Permanent coloring sinks into the hair shaft. It doesn't wash out. It lasts until the hair grows out. Tinted—colored—hair needs touching up about every four weeks, especially at the roots.

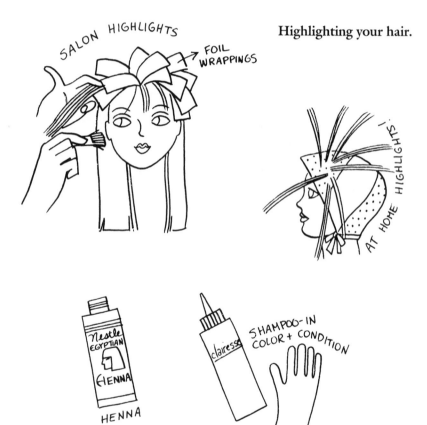

Highlighting your hair.

SALON HIGHLIGHTS

FOIL WRAPPINGS

AT HOME HIGHLIGHTS

Nestle EGYPTIAN HENNA

HENNA

clairesse

SHAMPOO-IN COLOR + CONDITION

STREAKING, PAINTING, TIPPING, AND FROSTING. All of these add highlights. But only a few strands are bleached, rather than the whole head. If this is done well, it looks natural. It looks almost as if the sun did the work.

Get Set

There's no need to accept the hair color you were born with if you'd like another. But if you're really thinking of a change from your natural color . . .

• Consult an expert for advice. The last thing you want is to damage your hair.

• Make sure the color you choose looks believable. Let it bring out the best in you. Good color will go well with your skin tone and play up your top features.

• Remember that the darker you are to begin with and the lighter you want to become, the more time and money you'll have to spend to keep the hair color up. It's wise to select a shade that's fairly close to your own natural color. If you're thinking about a bigger change, try on a wig in the new color. How do you look?

Start Rolling

Have you decided to color your hair yourself? The big plus is that it's cheaper. Finding an easy-to-use color kit is no problem at all. There are a lot of them on the market. Once you choose one, follow some basic rules.

Read the directions carefully and follow them to the letter.

Even if you've tinted your hair before, always do a patch test. You'll find out if your skin dislikes the product you have chosen. Prepare a small amount of coloring. Apply with a cotton stick inside an under arm crease. Leave on for twenty-four hours, being careful not to wash it away. If there's no skin reaction, it's okay to paint, streak, or color your hair.

If your hair has been recently permed, wait a few weeks before you color. All chemical treatments will cause changes in your hair. If the treatments are over-done, they will damage your hair.

Curl Up

If you don't have naturally curly hair, and you want to look as if you do, a *perm* can do the trick. A perm is a

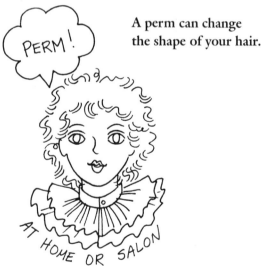

A perm can change the shape of your hair.

method of changing the shape of the hair with chemicals. First, a solution breaks down the chemical bonds of the hair. Next, rods bend the hair into a new shape. Last, the neutralizer locks curl in. Depending on the size of the rods, you can get most looks you're after. The smaller the rods are, the tighter the curl. The shape and direction the rods are rolled will also determine the look. However, the longer hair is, the less curly it will be. Permed or not, weight pulls hair down.

Before a perm, get a good haircut to insure an even curl. If you are planning to give yourself a home permanent, try a test curl to see how your hair takes it. Read the instructions carefully. After the perm, don't wash your hair for a few days. Then use a mild shampoo and apply a deep conditioner.

A perm is not recommended if you have allergies or sensitive skin. It is also not a good idea if your hair is damaged. A perm will dry hair out further.

How permanent is a perm? Some loosen up in a month. Others last until the hair is cut. Most last four to six months.

A body wave is a type of perm. It is an extremely loose perm. It gives hair added volume and fullness.

Relax It

If you have lots of too curly hair, you can straighten your locks. But be forewarned: This is a harsh thing to do to your hair. When straightening at home, use *extreme* caution. Follow directions. Straighten only new growth, not previously straightened hair. About every six to eight weeks, you'll need a touch-up. Always allow plenty of time between straightening and coloring your hair.

Relaxed hair needs extra-special care. The process robs the hair of both proteins and moisture. If you choose to relax your hair, condition it often. Have the ends cut frequently. Brush and comb hair gently.

8

Head In The Right Direction

Your hair is what you eat. The kind of hair you have depends a great deal on your diet. A poor diet can leave your hair limp, brittle, and dull. Even though hair can't run a temperature, it can look sick. Only a well-balanced diet can provide the nourishment your hair needs to grow healthy. Hair is nourished from the inside out.

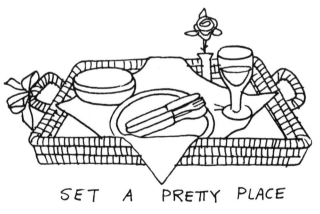

SET A PRETTY PLACE

Take time to eat properly.

Food for healthy hair.

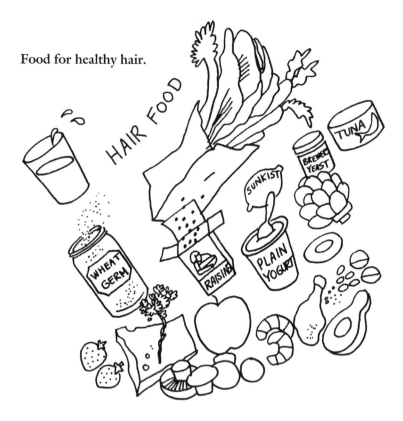

Everything we eat belongs in one of four food groups. Hair is 97 percent protein. It suffers when you cut protein intake. This means that lean meats, poultry, and fish should be on your daily menu. If you cut down on fruits and vegetables, your body will use your protein intake to do the job of delivering energy. Again it can make your hair look sick.

Don't skip meals or eat on the run. Sit down and let your body store the foods you take in. Exercise is also important. So is rest. With a healthy dose of both, you'll feel better. You'll help your hair look its best too.

9

Guard Against The Weather

Everybody talks about the weather. What you need is to do something about it. When the weather changes, so does your hair. You need a new hair care plan.

Beat The Heat

The lazy days of summer can give your hair a hard time. Heat from the sun can scorch hair. It can make your hair frizzy and dry. On rainy or humid days, hair absorbs extra moisture. This can make it look limp. Wind can also cause damage. And air conditioning dries out even the healthiest hair.

If you're going to be outdoors, cover your head with a hat. Protect your hair from too much sun. This may lighten its color and cause it to break. Without protection, tinted or bleached hair may turn orange.

Daily shampooing is also a summertime must. Scalp pores tend to open from the heat. This invites dirt and

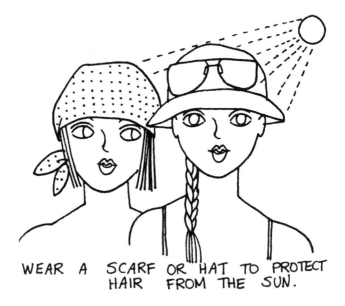

WEAR A SCARF OR HAT TO PROTECT HAIR FROM THE SUN.

dust. Heat also causes more oil production. Oily hair needs more sudsings. Try switching shampoos, if the one you're using isn't doing the trick.

Give your hair a weekly deep conditioning treatment to put moisture back in. Then use an instant conditioning creme on hair ends. You might try putting it on your hair before leaving for the beach.

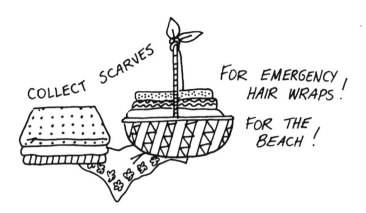

COLLECT SCARVES

FOR EMERGENCY HAIR WRAPS!

FOR THE BEACH!

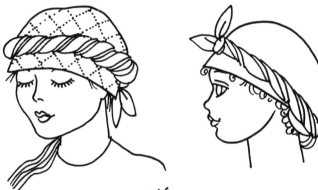

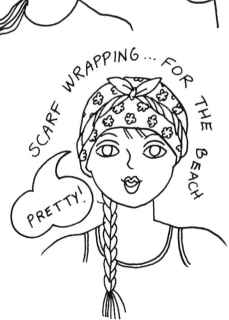

SCARF WRAPPING... FOR THE BEACH

PRETTY!

Whether you're a serious swimmer or a dog paddler, always shampoo and rinse the seawater or chlorine out of your hair. Do this as soon as you get out of the water. Both are hard on the hair. If you neglect to rinse them out, your hair may change color.

Adopt a neat summer hairdo. If you're wearing shoulder-length hair loose, put it up in a braid. If you like to tie your hair back, make sure you don't always tie it back in the same place. Also, don't tie it too tightly. That weakens hair. Always parting your hair in the same place can lead to a painful sunburn on your scalp.

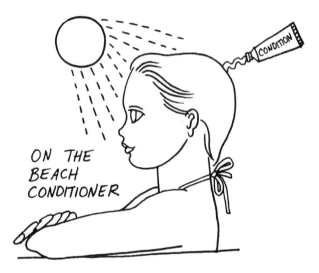

ON THE
BEACH
CONDITIONER

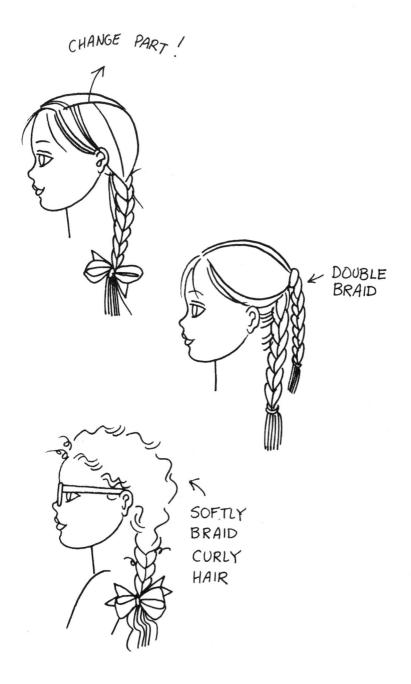

CHANGE PART!

DOUBLE
BRAID

SOFTLY
BRAID
CURLY
HAIR

Weather The Winter

Cold air is dry air. On cold winter days humidity often drops. When there's less moisture in the air, the air robs you of water. Hair suffers from winter dryness as skin does. Rough treatment from the wind can make matters worse. So can an overheated room. It can turn almost any head of hair into straw.

The only way to prevent hair from drying out is to winterize it. Keep hair covered in cold or windy weather. Combat static electricity by using a mild, mild shampoo. Also, don't use a hot blow dryer. Your hair will be the winner!

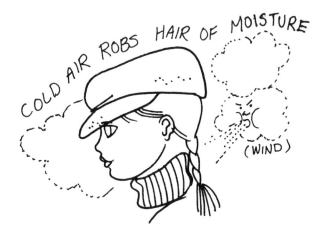

COLD AIR ROBS HAIR OF MOISTURE

(WIND)

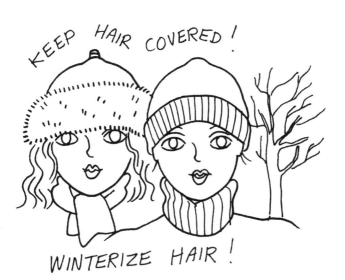

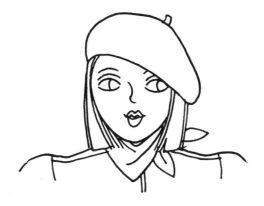

Protect your hair in cold weather.

Index

Baby shampoo, 25
Black hair, 13, 43-44
Bleaching, 22, 64, 65, 72
Blondes, 13, 21
Blow drying, 11, 40, 50-52
Body, 31
Braids, 75
Breakage, 14, 15
Brunettes, 13
Brush, brushing, 35, 36, 46-50

Chlorinated water, 11
Clairol hotline, 45
Coarse hair, 19, 20, 21
Cold, 11, 23, 24, 76-77
Color, hair, 11, 13, 21
Coloring, 22, 63-66
Comb, combing, 34-36, 46-50
Combination hair, 39-40
Conditioners, 21, 29-34, 37, 39,
    44, 72
Consultation, 60-61
Cortex, 10-11
Creme rinse, 29-30
Curling, 11, 52-54
Curly hair, 11, 12, 21
Cuticle, 10-11, 26, 29, 31, 32

Damage, hair, 11, 14-15, 18, 22,
    25, 30, 35, 42
Dandruff, 17, 40-42
Deep conditioning, 31-34, 44, 72
Diamond face, 59
Diet, 7, 13, 21, 22, 37, 69-70
Dry hair, 11, 18, 23, 24, 25, 30,
    31, 37-38, 71, 76

Egg conditioner, 31, 32
Exercise, 7, 70

Face shape, 55-59
Fine hair, 19, 21
Follicle, 11-13, 21, 22
Frizzies, 11, 18, 71
Frosting, 65

Gray hair, 11
Greasies, 17
Growth rate, 7, 13-14

Hair spray, 42
Hair styles and cuts, 55-62
Hairdressers, 60-62
Hats, 71-73, 76-77
Heart-shaped face, 57
Highlights, 63-65
Hot rollers, 50, 52
Humidity, 71, 76

Long hair, 27, 29, 48, 50
Loss, normal hair, 13-14

Medulla, 10-11
Melanin, 11
Moisture, 9-10, 11, 24, 71, 72

Natural bristle brush, 47-48
Natural conditioners, 31-32
Normal hair, 13-14, 18, 19, 23,
    25
Number, hair, 13

Oblong face, 58
Oil bath, 38, 39
Oil glands, 12, 17, 36
Oily hair, 17-18, 23, 25, 30, 36-37, 72
Oval hair, 55-56

Papilla, 13
Parts of the hair, 10-13
Pear-shaped face, 58
Perms, 22, 66-67
Peroxide, 64
Ponytail strain, 15
Processed hair, 22, 45
Protein, 9, 26, 31, 70

Redheads, 13
Relaxed hair, 22, 67-68
Rest, 7
Rinse, 28-29, 74
Rollers, 20, 52-54
Roots, 11-13
Round face, 57

Salt intake, 37
Scalp, 17, 27, 48
Scarves, 73
Sets, 20, 44, 52-54
Shampoo, 23-29, 36, 37, 39, 40, 41, 44, 72

Short hair, 27
Split ends, 18, 42
Square face, 56
Static electricity, 18, 19, 48, 76
Straight hair, 11, 12
Straightening, 22, 67-68
Streaking, 65
Stress, 37
Stretch test, 30-31
Styling, 20, 44, 52-54
Summer, 13, 71-75
Sun, 11, 24, 71-75
Swimming, 74

Tangles, 27, 28, 29, 30, 34, 43, 50
Texture, 7, 11, 19-20, 48
Thick hair, 21
Thin hair, 21, 40
Tipping hairdressers, 62
Towel drying, 34
Trimming, 42
Type, hair, 11-12, 16-19

Wavy hair, 11, 12
Weather, 11, 24, 71-77
Wind, 11, 71, 76
Winter, 11, 23, 24, 76-77

About the Author

Betty Lou Phillips grew up in Chagrin Falls, Ohio, where she showed registered quarterhorses, played tennis, and watched baseball, before attending Syracuse University in New York. After graduation, she taught in the Shaker Heights (Ohio) Public School System, married, and began a family. As her children's interest in sports expanded, so did her's, and Ms. Phillips became a sportswriter for *The Cleveland Press* and a special features editor for *Pro Quarterback,* a monthly. She has also written many articles and a number of books on various sports and other subjects. Ms. Phillips lives with her husband, John Roach, in Houston, Texas.